# Faecal Incontinence

is it really IBS?

A practical guide to discovering the true problem and getting the right help.

by
T R Lewis

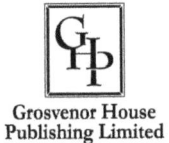

Grosvenor House
Publishing Limited

All rights reserved
Copyright © T R Lewis, 2015

The right of T R Lewis to be identified as the author of this
work has been asserted by him in accordance with Section 78
of the Copyright, Designs and Patents Act 1988

The book cover picture is copyright to T R Lewis

This book is published by
Grosvenor House Publishing Ltd
28-30 High Street, Guildford, Surrey, GU1 3EL.
www.grosvenorhousepublishing.co.uk

This book is sold subject to the conditions that it shall not, by way of
trade or otherwise, be lent, resold, hired out or otherwise circulated
without the author's or publisher's prior consent in any form of binding or
cover other than that in which it is published and
without a similar condition including this condition being imposed
on the subsequent purchaser.

A CIP record for this book
is available from the British Library

ISBN UK: 978-1-78148-476-0

In fond memory of

Evelyn Segal

1929 - 2015

# Index

| | |
|---|---|
| Preface | vii |
| Introduction: | ix |
| My story | 1 |
| The anatomy, and physiology, of continence | 18 |
| What exactly is IBS? | 27 |
| Take this to your GP. | 33 |
| Bristol Stool Chart | 39 |
| Your Doctor's Surgery | 42 |
| What tests might or should be done. | 48 |
| Biofeedback. | 65 |
| The emotional and psychological impact. | 72 |
| Coping with 'it' day to day. | 81 |
| Dietary issues | 89 |
| Sacral Nerve Stimulation | 94 |
| Epilogue | 98 |

# Preface

I'd never thought of writing a book and had I, I would certainly have liked to start it with something along the lines of ...once upon a time. This story however is no fairytale, in fact it's more like a horror story.

In short I was diagnosed with IBS when I was in my mid twenties. I had had some episodes of uncontrollable faecal incontinence already. I blindly accepted a diagnosis of IBS (Irritable Bowel Syndrome), initially no tests were done, not even a digital examination of my rear passage. The next twenty five or so years of my life were, at times, hell because of my inability to control my bowels. Then a chance meeting, with the son of a dear friend, Professor Tony Segal, changed my life.

It wasn't IBS, it had never been IBS and as a result I'd realistically gone twenty five years without any treatment, or at best with limited or incorrect treatment attempts.

In those twenty five years I've gained a large amount of knowledge on what should be done to ensure an accurate diagnosis is reached. If you're reading this book then chances are you are a sufferer. I hope this book will help prevent you from falling into the same misdiagnosis black hole that engrossed me.

# Introduction

What prompted me to write this book is the fear that what happened to me may be happening to others right now. I'm not saying that everyone who reads this book will find the cure for their problem, but I'm hoping that along the way some will gain from my experience and push to get the investigations done that will determine the exact cause of their symptoms. You should have hope that there is something that can be done for you as there are options available, but only if you know what is wrong with you in the first place.

It's important to remember that regardless of how minor, or how severe your particular problem is, or how long you've suffered with it, few GPs, your first port of call, are equipped with the specialist knowledge to investigate faecal incontinence thoroughly. I'm not having a dig at GPs, far from it I think they are great, but you just can't expect them to have the depth of knowledge a specialist has spent many additional years gaining.

Sadly my experience shows me that many gastroenterologists (who one would think should have the knowledge) are not 100% up to speed on this topic either. Are you even aware that there are doctors, and nurses, who specialise in incontinence? I was most certainly not aware of it until recently. Over the years I saw five GP's, three gastroenterologists, two psychologists, two acupuncturists and a psychiatrist (it sounds like a song!) before finally, by chance, meeting the man who saw past the hand-me-down diagnosis of Irritable Bowel Syndrome (IBS). It took him about five minutes to diagnose my main problem which was nothing at all to do with IBS. He referred me to St Mark's Hospital in Harrow (London, England), which is a centre of excellence for all things bowel. I finally received the thorough investigations that needed to be undertaken to discover that my problem was actually part physical, part dietary and part endorcrinal.

Faecal incontinence is debilitating, it affects every part of your life. It causes social isolation, lowers self esteem, may cause depression and, for me, left me exhausted and drained for much of my younger life. Bowel habits are scarcely dinner table conversation so you will rarely, if ever, hear people talking about it. You may well think that you are the only one with this problem or that there can't be many others with the problem. Well, you're wrong! The NHS (National Health Service) published guidelines in 2007 that state that between 1% and 10% of the UK population suffer with faecal incontinence and the National Institute of Health in the US estimated that in America there is somewhere in the region of eighteen million people known to have faecal incontinence. I say 'known' because faecal incontinence is one of the most under reported and therefore undiagnosed conditions. That makes sense, we see it as shameful, disgusting and the thought of an adult pooing their pants, like a baby, is horrific. The last thing most people will do is talk about it.

Faecal incontinence affects both sexes of all ages although more women are affected than men. In the elderly faecal incontinence is a major reason for institutionalisation as both the sufferer, and their families, find the condition extremely hard to live with. The loss of dignity, regardless of age or gender is impactful. Faecal incontinence may be a minor nuisance to you or, if it is severe, it may be a tragedy for you; your lifestyle may alter dramatically. Fear of embarrassment makes some sufferers avoid sexual relations so the potential impact of this condition on relationships and families is wide reaching.

Given the degree of embarrassment associated with faecal incontinence many people avoid telling their doctors about it and few, if any, GPs think to question patients about their continence. As a result the circle of silence is maintained, the condition goes undiagnosed, untreated, and people suffer needlessly.

Please don't think this book is intended to replace your doctor, it's not, but I do hope it will give you a sound basis for starting a constructive dialogue with them and possibly even prompt them to investigate you a little more thoroughly.

*Had I known what I know now my life would have been completely different*

*BUT remember everything that happens to you makes you who you are.*

*If you like yourself then perhaps this was all a life enhancing experience.*

# My story

I was born in 1965 in London. In 1966 my parents decided to emigrate to Australia. Mother all too frequently delights in entertaining others with the story of my nappy rash on the flight; looking back I now wonder if that was an omen of things to come!

I recall (I was just twenty or so), finding it hard to urinate without opening my bowels or at least being seated on the toilet to allow me to be able to open them if needed. I always had to use a cubical as standing at the urinal to go made me instantly want to open my bowels. The relaxing of my urethral sphincter, to allow the urine to pass, seemed to trigger a need to defecate. I got a little ribbing about it from friends but just shrugged it off as I'd had a lot worse than that over the years. Being a classical music loving male child growing up in the suburbs of Sydney lent itself to more than a fair share of bullying. Though I think in those days, the 70's and 80's, 'bullying' was all part of a thing called 'growing up'. With hindsight this was a clear signal that something was wrong down-below but it didn't seem serious at the time so I thought no more of it.

I moved back to London in 89 and was having a whale of time in the exciting and vibrant city lights. I got a job in a large department store (Harrods) and was doing really well in terms of progressing up the ladder. My life was just fun! The only stress I could honestly say I was under was that of trying to get up the said ladder. I'm a very positive person so I thought I was rather thriving on the pressure and expectation.

The first time I was faecally incontinent came completely out of the blue. I lodged with a wonderfully colourful man, Peter, then in his mid sixties, who hosted dinner parties at least twice a week. The most interesting people would attend from all walks of life, cab drivers to judges. This particular evening we feasted on Herring in a sour cream source, pheasant in a garlic and herb butter, the pheasant was far too high for my taste, but interesting nonetheless, a wonderful creme burlee followed for dessert and then a cheese board to die for. I went to bed over fed and with perhaps one, small, glass of wine too many.

The next morning I woke up as usual and readied myself for work. Then I was out of the door, a quick dash, running late, to get onto the Piccadilly Line tube in the sweltering heat to be packed in with the herd of workers heading into London. I didn't even make it into the tube station when I had this sudden and uncontrollable urge to defecate. I ran back to the flat, thankfully Peter was already out. I made it into the bathroom, in fact into the bath, as my bowels completely opened. I was covered in poo, it was everywhere. My suit trousers were completely soaked and even my shirt tail was covered in brown, stinking defecate.

I was lucky I had made it into the bath so pulled off my trousers which resulted in there being poo all over my legs and socks. Those of you who've been through this will know all too well that as you remove your trousers and underwear the poo is wiped all the way down your legs, it's disgusting in the extreme, it felt horrible and I was overcome with a sense of disgust and bewilderment. I turned on the shower and just stood there, semi clothed, soaking wet, covered in poo and surrounded by the foul smell.

"It must have been the pheasant" I thought, I'd never eaten high game before so that must have been it.

I cleaned myself up, called the manager of the department, from the land-line, no mobiles in those days, and explained that I had been ill but would be in shortly. I duly did but was anxious all the way to work. That happy little moment over life continued on as usual and all seemed fine down below. Fine, but I noticed that was getting an upset stomach quite often. Then it happened again, this time I had stayed the night at a friend's bedsit, not far from home. It was one of those student accommodation situations in which the toilet and bathroom are shared by many.

There was only one toilet and my friend was in it when the urge came over me again. Panic filled me, what could I do? He had just gone in the loo and clearly was going to be there for a while. I could feel things coming and was clenching my buttocks as hard as I possibly could but I was losing the battle. I finally saw a waste paper basket in the corner of the room so squatted over it and let go. The full contents of my bowel, under pressure and stinking, went into the bin. Needless to say there was no toilet paper to hand so I just stood there like a baby with a dirty bottom; I think with hindsight I was in shock. I dressed immediately, dirty bum and all, and waited for my friend to return. The minutes seemed like hours.

I don't think I've ever been so embarrassed in my life. He came back into his own room to a wall of stench, the stench of human defecate. There I was, next to a bin of my own poo, and all I could do was apologise. I couldn't offer any reason to him other than to say that I was sorry, that I just couldn't hold it in. The poo was leaking from the plastic bag lining the bin so I took the whole thing and ran home.

It was at this point that I decided to go to the doctor. I explained to him that I'd had some problems with my tummy, to be completely fair to him I didn't tell him I'd been catastrophically incontinent, I just said something like 'I'd had a couple of accidents'. He didn't ask me to define 'accidents', I wasn't asked to lie down, he didn't examine me in any way, not even a digital examination of my back passage nor did he ask any questions to determine a history of my usual bowel habits. I know it's very easy to criticize now but come on, a man in his early twenties walks in saying he's completely fit and healthy but has 'had a couple of accidents' can't be an everyday occurrence. Well, you guessed it, 'you've got IBS!' that was it, done, dusted. He gave me a prescription for Colofac tablets, which are an antispasmodic, and I left.

From then on things gradually went downhill, I'd have good days and bad days. Good days would mean something like only going to the toilet to defecate say four times in the day. Bad days it would be anything up to ten or even more times in a day. I started filling my underwear with toilet paper carefully layered to form a sort of make-shift panty liner. The 'help' from that was more psychological than practical.

Gradually the years passed and I muddled by. Getting to work on the tube became impossible because I feared being stuck in the tube if I had another accident, and there were many accidents during those years. Not always catastrophic accidents but no fun regardless. One unfortunately memorable tube journey involved coming all the way from East London to West London when it happened. I spent the whole journey standing with my back to the wall in fear that I have leaked onto my jeans. My poker-face got tested to the limits on that trip, however the smell I fear gave me away. After this I decided that I had to move close enough to work to be able to walk in so my journey developed into a loo hopping exercise. I'd leave the flat and if I was bad I would stop at the public convenience about 70 meters away. That would then see me straight until the next loo which was on the other side of the park about 20 minutes away with a peaceful pace. But 'peaceful pace' soon gave way to a 'desperate dash' as the adrenaline kicked in. I now realise I was training myself, like Pavlov and his dogs, to panic. I would be totally focused on what my gut was doing and without fail it would trigger at a certain point along the journey. That in turn would flick my adrenaline switch, the adrenaline would flow which in turn increases gut motility, wham bam, run to the loo. If the loo wasn't open the bushes sufficed regardless of the weather.

From there it was another dash to McDonald's before finally into the store (Harrods), staff loos, second door on the left after you signed in; I could have done it blindfolded. Once in the building I was usually Okay because I knew where the toilets were and I would move around the store following pre-planed routes that I knew would have me near a loo quickly if required. I would later understand the irony of this; panic attacks only come when you are out of your comfort zone. Having the routes planned was in itself a comfort zone.

Going home was never as bad. I now know that it was because I was more in control of the adrenaline, less panic because if I did have an accident I was going home and could deal with it there in safety; less pressure, less adrenaline. Going out socially was really difficult as I was on constant alert for the toilets. Staying away at friends homes was next to impossible unless I could ascertain if I would have my own toilet; it became easier to simply refuse the invitation automatically. Speaking of going out, you sufferers will know that you can spot a loo the second you walk into a place. No matter where you are or what you're doing, the prime focus of your mind is to find the loo. As you walk along the street you'll be clocking the pubs, fast food places, coffee shops etc. Public toilets are almost a thing of the past but you'll always have a coin ready in case you come across one of those automatic loos on the street. Faecal incontinence is a full time job, the only real rest you get from being on loo patrol is when you are at home, or asleep. It hasn't been until recently that I have realised how draining that whole process was.

With the move of house came a new GP, a female this time so I was more open, crazy I know, but it's true. She was sympathetic and sent me to a gastroenterologist at one of the private hospitals. He did put his finger up my bum so that was a step in the right direction. He also ordered some blood tests and a Sigmoidoscopy (a small camera inserted into the back passage – described in more detail later in the book).

The Sigmoidoscopy preparation involved an enema just prior to the procedure. Okay, no problem I thought,

I'll be in a hospital situation so plenty of loos around. I duly arrive and am asked to change into a gown. The procedure room annex ward had six beds, we were all there for the same sort of thing so six enemas went flying that morning. ONE TOILET. Do I need to go on? One toilet, occupied most of the time by one of my five post-enema friends and me with my enema in full swing. Fortunately the floors were vinyl.

So, I'm off back to see the Gastroenterologist who tells me that there is nothing wrong in my Sigmoid colon but he stops there. No further test. He does however introduce me to a) a psychologist and b) my new best friend, Imodium (Loperamide). Imodium really did help me enormously and for this I must be grateful, I only wish I'd bought shares and that he'd bothered to tell me how to take it.

The psychologist was a different matter. I spent several hours learning to breathe deeply, a complete waste of time. She also told me that they were now experimenting, and had had good results with, antidepressants. She prescribed, via the gastroenterologist, Seroxat which is used for anxiety disorders, depression and panic disorder. I took this but it had almost no effect at all on the symptoms. As the weeks past she finally realised that things were not improving. She then sent me on to her mentor, with whom she was working on a study about the use of antidepressants in cases, of diarrhoea predominant IBS, such as mine, in Harley Street. He was a psychiatrist, a lovely man that I liked a great deal. He did however raise an eyebrow in dismay when he discovered she had me on Seroxat. He said in the most professional way that it was completely the wrong drug. Brilliant I thought, now we're getting somewhere.

If it's the wrong drug then he clearly knows what the right drug is.

Anafranil: So here we are I'm now on the right drug, I assumed at the right dose, but I'm almost falling asleep at work, sweating buckets for no reason, and by this stage I'd moved jobs and was running the whole company so this was just not an option. On top of that my libido diminished drastically and it was virtually impossible for me to climax; not a great situation for a man in the prime of his sexual life. Again the weeks and months went on but, despite the side affects, no improvement with my stomach and still episodes of faecal incontinence. So it was time for the next gastroenterologist, a friend of the psychiatrist and also in Harley Street. This one a professor no less. I liked him too, if fact I've liked all of my doctors. First thing he says is that the dosage of Anafranil I'm on is way too high (um didn't the last guy raise an eyebrow at the other dosage? – are you getting confused yet?) so he reduced it by 75%. He decided that he would rethink everything and get to the bottom of this problem; I was delighted and relieved. So more tests, this time much more thorough and a barium meal too (so gross). Everything was, once again clear. I stayed under his care, with no improvement, for years.

By this time the internet was around and I, like so many others, was searching it for the miracle cure. I discovered on one of the US IBS sites, remember at this point they were all still saying it was diarrhoea predominant IBS, that people had been having great success with a new antidepressant called Zyban. Trouble is that Zyban is the stop smoking drug and is not registered for use with IBS here in the UK. Professor Gastro-Man kindly wrote to my GP and asked him (yes I'd changed surgery again) to offer this to me. I must say that it really did help, it seemed to slow things down a little and gave the stools a chance to sort of form, at least sometimes. I still had good and bad days, my stools were occasionally formed but certainly never 'normal' stools unless I was dosed to the eyeballs with Imodium, which would make me feel nauseous so a catch twenty two. By this stage I'd moved on to ladies panty liners and accepted that when I was away on business I would just have to dose up on the Imodium and cope the nausea. (I would later discover that the Imodium was not the cause of the nausea.) Alone in my hotel room I'd sometimes cry.

Yet more years went on and I tried acupuncture, which I believe in fully, just ask my cat (but that's another story). It really helped me sleep but did nothing for the tummy. I did try the Chinese herbs but wow that was a big mistake, serious faecal incontinence incident following that. Sleep was something that I could never get enough of, nothing to do the with antidepressants that I remained on for years but I was drained all of the time. I put that down to losing all the nutrients that my body was not absorbing as the food was rushing through my system. I could see, in the toilet bowl, that the food wasn't being digested properly. I complained to Professor Gastro-Man that I had much wind and mucus coming out but this he said was just the way it is with IBS.

By this time I'm in my mid forties and I'm on the big guns, Attends disposable incontinence pads and full on disposable adult nappies. We went to Australia to visit my parents. Mother had no idea that I was back in nappies, at least this time there was no rash.

Things are now really bad, in fact they are getting considerably worse as I age, I've had some serious faecal incontinence catastrophes and the panic attacks are coming thick and fast. Even going to the corner shop is an issue. I had to prepare for every step outside of the safety zone that is home. I'd had two catastrophic incidents at Heathrow airport within three months of each other. The second time, having cleaned up and changed in to my replacement clothes (I always carried spares) I simply had to abandon the whole trip. The thought of sitting, probably smelling, on the flight and then having to rush to the hotel to shower in advance of the meetings was too much for me. I explained to the airport authorities that I was ill and they had me escorted from the terminal back into public space. Each time I'd go back to Harley Street it's the same old story, front up, talk for a bit then 'sorry old chap this is just your lot in life'. Somehow I've managed to keep positive throughout all of this, Lord knows how, but there have certainly been times when I've crawled under the duvet.

Life sometimes offers up a quirky turn or two, mine was befriending a great lady in her eighties. We played piano duets together and got on like a house on fire. One day she came to the vet to collect the aforementioned cat and you guessed it, panic attack in the car, quick, I need a story and I need a loo NOW!. I managed one of the standard excuses, "think I ate something bad, we had takeaway last night and my partner is not well either" etc. Off I run to Costa Coffee and thankfully managed to get to the loo without an accident. On returning to the car she, with the wisdom of age, quizzed me and I confessed. I told her that I have this awful problem, the urgency and so on. She was great, she said she too suffers with something similar and she knew exactly how I felt. That was great in itself, just having someone from outside knowing was a real relief. (Other than my partner only one other very close friend knew about it.) Her reaction made it much easier for me to tell other friends, who too, were all great. My partner knew of course and was incredibly helpful and supportive. I hate to think how many hours of that life were wasted waiting outside of toilets.

Here's the wonderful bit.

My octogenarian friend's son is a Professor of Crohn's disease at UCL (University College London). She insisted that I went to see him as she felt sure that he would be able to help me. Well not to look a gift horse in the mouth, and having gotten a grand total of nowhere with the previous crews over twenty odd years, I decided to go. It took him about five minutes of questioning to come up with the diagnosis. He asked questions like; Is there a lot of mucus, wind?; Are you bloated?; Has anyone checked for dietary issues like a wheat allergy? ('not knowingly' was the answer). Then the bomb shell…'I don't think you've got IBS, I think you're lactose intolerant'. Well I'd not heard that one before.

I was instructed to stop lactose (cow's milk, butter etc) completely and to let him know in 24 hours if I'd improved. It was like a magic wand had been waved. No lactose at all, and it's hard because it's hidden in so many products, but I had stools! real ones, not solid but not the watery mush that I'd had for all those years. It was a miracle.

He did however suspect that this was not the sole reason for the problem as it didn't explain the faecal incontinence, it explained why I was getting the loose stools and urgency – the body working frantically to expel the lactose (why the other two gastroenterologists didn't make that same simple connection will forever remain, a very worrying, mystery). So I was sent off to the third gastroenterologist, again a lovely man. He did all the tests again but this time I had a new ones. An anal ultrasound along with sphincter strength tests and a defecography scan (I describe the tests later for you). The ultrasound test was embarrassing but not painful, as was the strength tests. I didn't know it at the time but the key tests for me were the defecography and the endo-anal ultrasound. For the defectography I was filled from the rear with barium meal paste to the point where I felt I could no longer hold it. The doctor told me that when I got to that point to let him know and then I was to sit on a commode in the middle of the room and poo myself, on their command, for the x-ray camera. What fun!

Well, the lovely assistant was new and didn't quite know how to work the equipment. I was sitting on the commode and he was asking me to hold on until he could work out how to get the machine to work. Naturally I started a panic attack and then the heavens opened. I just couldn't hold it anymore. I was being told, firmly, to hold on but I couldn't, no matter how hard I tried I just couldn't. I started screaming, screaming in full voice, screaming in panic, screaming, "I can't, I can't!, this is what happens, I just can't!"

This was a truly humiliating experience for me. I felt that I had lost what remaining dignity I had. I was sitting on a loo seat in front of three people pooing myself. The technician was in panic as it was he that was messing it all up, I was in panic because I was pooing myself against my will and the lovely doctor and nurse where just standing there calmly, unmoved, watching this all unfold. It was hideous.

Looking on the bright side the doctor did manage to get enough footage to find the problem. He could see on the monitor that part of my internal anal sphincter simply wasn't working properly. It was like a donut with a bite missing. One very small section of the ring of muscle didn't work at all so no matter how hard it would squeeze itself it could never fully shut off the tube of bowel. In other words I was absolutely incapable, physically, of holding back my stools.

The doctor and I sat together quietly after I cleaned up. I was close to tears and he was extremely supportive. I have goose bumps just recalling the moment he told me that he knew what was wrong with me. All of these years, dozens of doctors' appointments, tests, drugs, accidents, panic attacks, feelings of disgust and shame and there it was, there really was a problem, it was the best gift anyone could ever have given me. He told me that there was an operation, implanting something that gives out an electric current, great results, almost a complete cure rate. I was too shocked to take in what he was saying, I just sat there welling up.

Now I'm chomping at the bit to see the third gastroenterologist again to find out what this operation thing is. Where do I sign, I'm in, how soon can you do it? He sat there and said, "oh yes I see. Now let's see how you get on without the lactose but with Imodium and come back and see me in three months!" I was gutted.

The weekly cup of tea with my dear octogenarian. I recounted all the news and she was infuriated. "He can't do that", " you must go back to see my son". Well I did go back and he did it again, another rabbit from the hat. He'd already done some research on it and immediately sent me to St Mark's to one of his colleagues from days gone by who specialises in Sacral Nerve Stimulators. This was the device that the radiographer had been referring to, a pacemaker for the bum as I think of him, I say him because I called him 'Harry', as in 'Harry Potter' – he's magical.

'Harry' is extremely expensive and works very well for most, but not for all. He also works better on the right side for some and the left side for others. Given the expense and to ensure that he is right for you, and to work out which side is best for you if he is, a temporary device is fitted for three weeks. This means an operation under general anaesthetic to insert two electrodes, right and left, along the sacral nerve at around the middle of the buttocks. An external power control unit is attached that one must keep on ones belt. During the three weeks trial no showers or baths are permitted, only washes at the sink, which is rather frustrating to say the very least. The first week one side is used and you monitor its impact on your symptoms at varying strengths. For the second week you switch to the other side and compare the results. In the final week you are able to use whichever side you prefer. For me the right side proved much more effective than the left. The electrode wires are removed from your buttocks in the doctors practice with no anaesthetic and it does not hurt at all. The first bath in three weeks is one of the most pleasurable memories of my life.

After the trial the doctor decides if 'Harry' is for you, if so you go back in some weeks later for another operation to fit the permanent device under your skin. It's about the size of a two euro coin and the scar about ten centre metres long. The device is controlled with a remote control unit on which you can increase or

FAECAL INCONTINENCE IS IT REALLY IBS?

decrease the amplitude of the electric pulse sent to the sacral nerve. You also have several programmes that send the pulse from different places on the wire that has been inserted along your sacral nerve.

'Harry' changed my life. A combination of no lactose at all and 'Harry' sending out his little electric pulse to block the 'I need to go' signals going up to my brain made a world of difference to me. I was vastly improved and things were going really well until some months in I had two episodes of faecal incontinence. I went back to the surgeon who passed me onto an incontinence specialist, a lady I now call the 'Goddess'. I had yet more tests, checking for nasty cancers and such like (which thankfully it wasn't) and finally my partner's beetroot soup gave the clue which pinned down the final piece of the jigsaw. On top of the lactose intolerance I have rapid gut transit. The soup was delicious but within one hour and forty five minuets of consuming it I was on the loo with bright red faecal matter all over the bowl. The Goddess sat with me and explained to me that we needed to slow my whole gut down to increase the time the food stays in my gut, she also told me, in detail, how to take Imodium; no one had ever done that before and it has been incredibly beneficial. I now take my Imodium 30 to 60 minutes before each meal, four x 2mg capsules in the morning, three at lunch and one before dinner. Imodium is a wonderfully safe drug but you must know how to use it. Simply taking it when you have a problem is of little use, closing the stable door after the horse has bolted, as it were. The Imodium has slowed my gut so that stools now form in a normal way. 'Harry' can now do exactly what he's meant to do because he needs a stool to be effective, he's not able to hold back water under pressure.

One rather annoying thing I've discovered is that many medications contain lactose added in the formation of the table/capsule themselves. I was gutted to see that my Imodium capsules contain lactose as does one other of my medications. At this stage there is nothing I can do to avoid that, and the amounts are tiny, but I'm keeping an eye on it every time I go into a Pharmacy, as things/brands do change.

So twenty five years down the line I don't use incontinence pads, I don't eat lactose and I lead an almost normal life. I'm still working on some of the hang-over issues from all those years of panic attacks but, with the help of a hypnotherapist I'm doing incredibly well and I can soon see a time when I'll be as close to normal as someone with a malfunctioning sphincter can be.

Had I been investigated properly from the start I would have lead a very different life. Granted the SNS implant is relatively new but I would a have known that there was a physical problem and could have avoided years of drugs that I simply did not need. The main thing would have been knowledge, just knowing I had a problem would have been a huge help but as it was I just thought it was me. I lived with a cloud over me for all those years, and a pretty big one if I'm honest.

*So that's enough about me. Let's move on to working out what might be wrong with you.*

# The anatomy, and physiology, of continence

Thankfully most people never have to give continence a second thought. They function on a day-to-day basis without ever needing to give even a passing thought to whether they will foul their underwear or whether they shouldn't involve themselves in certain activities or place themselves in certain situations because they may have an accident. It would never occur to them that they might have an accident that is so profound that people around them would notice either the smell, or worse, the soiling of their clothes. Sadly a not so small number of us do have to think about this sort of thing, and think about it constantly. It prevents some from leaving their homes for work and I'm sure many of us have missed important social events because we were simply too scared to risk the embarrassment of an accident.

I think it is wise for you to understand what should happen in 'normal' continence before we go any further. If you understand what should happen then hopefully you, with the help of your doctors, will be able to work out what is not happening in your individual case.

Remember faecal incontinence is not a disease or illness, it is a symptom which represents a malfunction in one of the intricate interactions that take place between the muscles and the brain that, combined, maintain continence. It may not be simply a malfunction with one of the muscles. There is a highly sophisticated ballet in action throughout your nervous system that sends and receives signals. These signals must occur at exactly the right moment within the sequence. If they don't, or there are other factors involved such as in my case with the lactose intolerance and rapid gut transit, you may lose continence. Let's start at the top:

We ingest our food via the mouth where it is masticated (chewed) in order to crush it and add saliva ready for it to start it's transit through the body. Once chewed we swallow, the now soft and wet mass called a bolus, into our oesophagus where the muscles in the wall of the oesophagus move it down into the stomach by a process of wave like motions call peristalsis.

When it reaches the stomach its strong muscles churn the food and mix it with acids and enzymes that continue the digestion process that began in the mouth. The food generally spends between one and three hours in the stomach. After that time it is a watery fluid that is then squeezed through into the small intestine where yet more churning and peristalsis move it along the many metres of gut. In a normal situation the food should be in the small intestine for between two and six hours.

Some of the watery fluid is absorbed by the body through the blood vessels lining the wall of the small intestine. The blood then takes the nutrients to the various parts of the body. What remains unabsorbed in the small intestine after these many hours is emptied into the much wider, but shorter, colon.

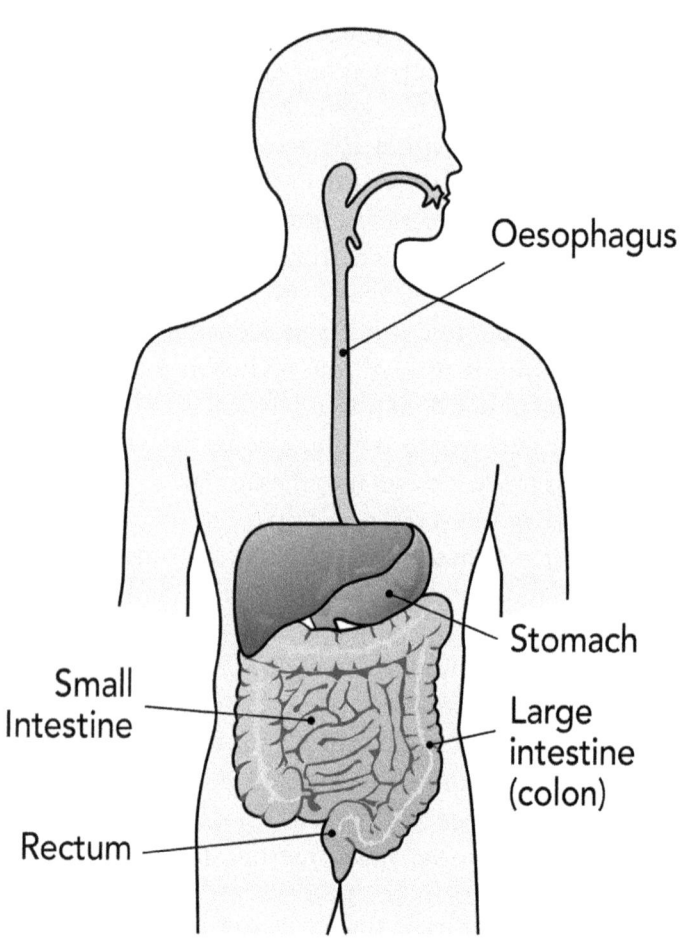

The colon works at a much slower pace than the small intestine and the remnants of the food will remain there for between twelve to forty eight hours.

In the colon much of the water content, and many of the minerals, are absorbed and the material gradually becomes more solid. As the material travels across the long section at the top of the colon (transverse colon) it becomes more formed – this material is then called faeces.

Contractions in the colon propel the stool down the descending section of the colon into the 'S' shaped sigmoid colon and rectum where it is further dehydrated and also stored. The colon and rectum are much more elastic than the small intestine and can therefore hold a large amount of faeces prior to defecation. In the rectum a solid column of stool is held ready for elimination. It is important that the stool moves slowly through the colon so that water can be absorbed and the stool formed. If the stool were to move too quickly then we would have great difficulty controlling our bowels, as when we have diarrhoea.

The formed stool sits in the rectum until we are full and the nervous system sends our brain the signal that we are ready to evacuate our bowels. The colon knows it is the right time because it senses the stretching as the rectum enlarges to hold the volume of the stool. Once we get the signal to go we take a conscious decision whether to go immediately or whether to wait for a more convenient time.

The anus is the final inch or so of the rectum. It is surrounded by the internal anal sphincter except at its very end, where it is surrounded by the external anal sphincter (the part we think of as our bottom).

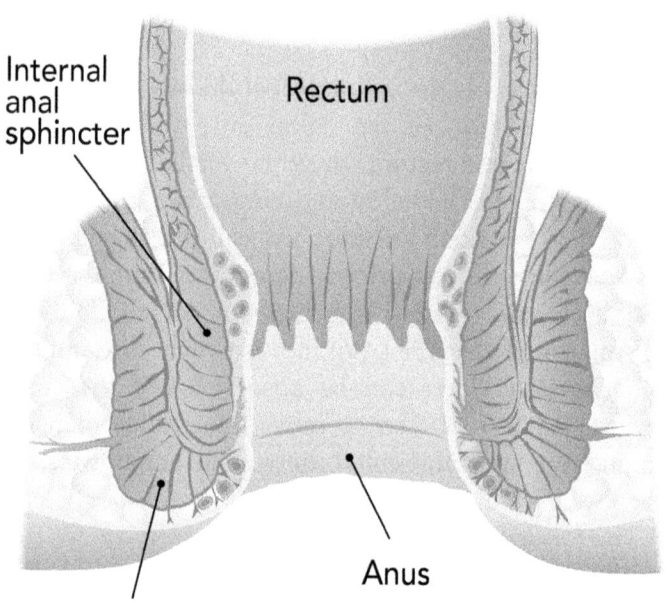

## FAECAL INCONTINENCE IS IT REALLY IBS?

The internal anal sphincter sits in a state of permanent contraction; that is its 'resting' position. It is rather like the mechanism that allows birds, and bats, not to fall from their respective perches when they are asleep; they have to stretch their muscles to open their feet which are 'resting' in the clenched position. The internal anal sphincter is permanently clenched like this in order to prevent any faeces, solid or liquid, from escaping from the rectum.

When enough faeces (stool) has built up in the rectum, and the rectal wall as stretched enough to trigger a signal, the clenched internal anal sphincter will automatically react to the pressure associated with the stretching of the wall, by opening up for a split second. This allows a small amount of faecal material down into the column just above, but not quite touching, the anus (your bottom), a test run as it were.

When we feel this sudden short rush heading towards the anus we automatically clench our external anal sphincter (bottom) to prevent an accident. We do this because we learned to do it when we were toilet trained. It has become an automatic reaction so we no longer even think about doing it, it all just happens.

Another split second later the internal anal sphincter clenches tight again forcing the small amount of material that was allowed down towards the anus back up into the rectum. It does this by squeezing tight from the lower end of the muscle and working back up. As all of that is happening signals are being sent up to your brain requesting instructions; "do you want to go now or wait?" If the response is 'wait' then the internal anal sphincter will remain clenched holding back the material until you decide to go on your terms; the sphincter is very strong and can hold off the stool for many hours if required. When you get to a toilet and are ready to evacuate your bowel the message to the internal anal sphincter will be 'open up'. As you have given the all clear signal to the internal anal sphincter your brain will automatically send a signal to the external anal sphincter (your bottom) to relax and allow the stool to pass from the body uninterrupted. The opening of the internal sphincter therefore automatically triggers the relaxing of the external sphincter; at that stage you no longer have 'manual' control of the external sphincter.

To summarize there are four basic elements involved in continence:

1) Your colon needs to be functioning properly so that it can store the faecal material.
2) A signal needs to be sent up to the brain from your internal anal sphincter saying "hey, what do you want me to do with this stool that's pushing on me?"
3) The brain needs to consider that question and send an instruction back to the sphincter telling it what to do either; 'hold on' or 'go'.
4) The two sphincters need to do their jobs <u>together</u> in order to hold back the faeces until the brain's answer is received.

As you can see the act of continence is a mix of muscles reacting automatically and voluntarily and, at the same time, a range of signals going to and from the muscles to your brain. If any one of these intricate factors fails, or even just gets out of sequence then incontinence will occur.

\*\*\*\*\*\*\*

For me the problem was the internal anal sphincter wasn't able to push the stool back up into the rectum after the 'test run' section of the continence ballet. The reason for that was two-fold, firstly the sphincter was not functioning correctly, so it was not able to contract fully (a donut with a bite missing), and secondly the faecal material was, because of the lactose intolerance and rapid gut transit, not formed into a solid stool. As a consequence the material would simply be moved around the space at the neck of the internal sphincter rather than being pushed back up into the rectum. The faecal material was also under pressure because my body saw the lactose as an unwanted foreign body and battled to expel it, with force, in the same way your body expels diarrhoea when you have an infection or poisoning in the gut. Therefore my internal sphincter was forced open by the faecal material that was under pressure and the external sphincter opened automatically as a direct result. Of course this resulted in me opening my bowels against my will whenever this series of mechanical triggers came into play. Add to that the impact of the adrenaline increasing the gut motility and it's safe to say these periods were far from fun for me.

*The IBS black hole...that last place you want to get stuck in.*

# What exactly is IBS

As I said in the introduction, I wrote this book in the hope that I could help to prevent others from falling in to what I call the IBS black hole. So often I read in the internet chat rooms that sufferers of faecal incontinence have been diagnosed with IBS and frequently, like with me, little or no investigation has been done to support that diagnosis or, more importantly, rule out the many other possible diagnoses.

IBS is technically a diagnosis however it is also a rather convenient umbrella diagnosis that is, unfortunately, sometimes issued without due consideration.

The Rome Criteria are the agreed current standard for the diagnosis of IBS but the UK's NICE (National Institute for Health and Care Excellence) guidelines sum it up in a simple A,B,C.

**A**bdominal pain or discomfort
**B**loating
**C**hange in bowel habits

Here is an overview of the Rome version:

The Rome diagnostic criteria of Irritable Bowel Syndrome always presumes the absence of a structural or biochemical explanation for the symptoms.

## The criteria are:

Irritable Bowel Syndrome can be diagnosed based on at least 12 weeks (which need not be consecutive) in the preceding 12 months, of *abdominal discomfort or pain that has two out of three of these features*:

1. Relieved with defecation; and/or
2. Onset associated with a change in frequency of stool; and/or
3. Onset associated with a change in form (appearance) of stool.

## Symptoms that Cumulatively Support the Diagnosis of IBS:

1. Abnormal stool frequency (may be defined as greater than 3 bowel movements per day or less than 3 bowel movements per week);
2. Abnormal stool form (lumpy/hard or loose/watery stool);
3. Abnormal stool passage (straining, urgency, or feeling of incomplete evacuation);
4. Passage of mucus;
5. Bloating or feeling of abdominal distension.

The trouble with being a sufferer of faecal incontinence is that you may well have IBS or some of the symptoms of IBS. What you must hold clear in your mind is that IBS does not explain faecal incontinence.

I'm going to say that again…

## IBS does not explain faecal incontinence.

In order to explain your own faecal incontinence you need to work out where and why your normal continence is failing. For example:

Haemorrhoids or polyps, at the level of the anal canal, may prevent normal function of the anal sphincter(s) by getting in the way and allowing liquid or loose stool material, that would normally be held back, to pass and exit the anus.

Mucus escaping and soiling underclothes may be the first sign of a prolapse.

Fistulas, like tunnels, may completely bypass the anus and deposit faecal material directly onto underwear.

Some people may have issues with the sensory nerves that must send, and receive, the messages to and from the brain. They may not know that their rectum is full, or may not realise that until it is too late for them to act on it in a normal way.

Others, like me, may have some malformation and may not be able to squeeze the sphincters tightly enough in order to retain the faecal material in place.

Diarrhoea, or a change in stool consistency, is often associated with faecal incontinence as it is much harder for us to hold back liquid/soft stool than solid formed stool. If your faecal incontinence is caused as a result of the colon madly trying to expel the diarrhoea/soft stool then you need to know what is causing that in the first place.

Diarrhoea is generally accepted to occur as a result of four mechanisms.

1) Increased secretion of fluid.
2) Reduced absorption of fluids.
3) Introduction of chemicals that increase the flow of fluid into the bowel.
4) Increased bowel movement.

Tests are available to determine if any of these factors are key in your particular problem. Discovering the answer to that question may well lead to the discovery that there is something else malfunctioning in the 'ballet' of the tummy.

One of the most common causes of faecal incontinence is damage to the anorectal muscles from surgical procedures such as haemorrhoidectomy or fistula repair. These procedures can leave scar tissue that hardens and prevents proper functioning of the anal muscles.

Women's anal muscles are at risk of tearing during childbirth or being damaged during episiotomy. In such cases it may take years (the muscles gradually weaken with age) before this damage causes faecal incontinence. Very often the women in question will not even be aware that this damage has occurred so there is no conscious link for them when their faecal incontinence appears.

Also what may appear to be a completely unrelated condition such as hyperthyroidism may in fact result in a weakness of the anorectal muscles.

You can see from this non-exhaustive list that there are many possible causes of faecal incontinence.

If, like me, you are simply told your problem is IBS and there is no further thought or tests then respectfully request that more investigation is done to rule out the other possibilities.

If you find yourself having to push or even fight your doctor to get these test done then it may be time to consider an alternative opinion with a doctor who is more open to the idea. Never lose sight of the fact that faecal incontinence is not caused by IBS, it is a separate and quite possibly completely unrelated problem.

*Get yourself ready...*

# Take this to your GP

You want to go to your doctor with as much information for them as possible. Simply telling them you are having accidents doesn't give them much to go on and the reality is that some doctors will not dig deeper to get to the root cause of the problem.

You want to have as much information about your condition to hand so before you go to the doctor keep a symptoms' diary for a few weeks (or days if you have a continuous problem) and take that with you.

Note in the diary;

- Whether or not you had urgency,
- What you were doing at the time,
- Were you under any stress,
- Were you out of your comfort zone,
- What you ate the day/evening before,
- Any non prescription drugs you took,
- How it made you feel,
- How did it affect those around you
- Every element of the situations you can think of.

Be very clear and concise with your doctor. Explain how your day-to-day functioning is affected. Stress to them that you do not wish to live with this problem if it is at all possible. Stress that you would like to ensure that all possible tests are done to ensure that you know exactly what is going on with your body.

This information along with the questions from the doctor will help to colour in the entire picture, both for them and, in many ways more importantly, for you. Had I been asked to do this I would have seen that my faecal incontinence was worse after the consumption of lactose and I'm sure I would have noted sooner that the food was rushing through my body at a vastly increased rate above normal.

When you go to the GP, if you feel comfortable to, take someone you trust with you. I assure you that having someone you can speak with freely is a real comfort. Having someone along side will help to ensure you don't miss anything the doctor says or asks you. Having been through all of this I can assure you that it is embarrassing and stressful; I'm sure I was not on top intellectual form at many of the various visits with the doctors. It's also really important not to withhold any information. I know you'll be embarrassed but do your best to complete the picture, no matter how small the details seems. There may be a clue in the very bit of information you don't pass on. That is why the symptoms diary is vital. Feel free to take notes or have your friend take notes, this is far too important to miss anything.

Your doctor will, or at least should, ask you things like:

1) How long can you hold on after the urge comes?
2) Does physical activity make you have an accident?
3) Do you have to strain when you go?
4) Is the any blood in the stool?

5) Do you have any cramps before or while going?
6) Do you feel that you have completely emptied yourself?
7) Have you noticed any connection with food and your bowel movements, their nature or frequency?
8) Have you travelled anywhere exotic recently?
9) Have you had any anal injury or surgery in that area?
10) Is there mucus with the stools?
11) Where are your stools on the Bristol Stool Chart? (more on that later)
12) Does it smell bad or more at some times than others?
13) Is there any pattern with your bowel habits?
14) Do you have large amounts of flatulence?
15) Are you able to clean yourself easily after evacuation?

Your doctor will also want to examine you externally to see if there are any areas of hardness in the gut, lumps in your glands, general soreness or any other abnormalities in or around your tummy area. They will also need to do an internal examination of the anus using their gloved and lubricated finger.

For women internal examinations are much more common and theoretically they should be more used to them. As a man I can tell you these types of exams are rare in your youth and psychologically quite distressing but, unless you want to spend the rest of your life in nappies, you just need to man up and accept it.

Following the medical history and physical examinations the doctor may be in a position to suggest a preliminary diagnosis. They should however confirm this diagnosis with one of more or the specialised diagnostic tests available. If there are not able to offer a preliminary diagnosis then they should refer you to a gastroenterologist for further tests. With hindsight, and assuming we'd had the internet in those days, I would have researched this thoroughly before going to the GP. With the head I have now on my shoulders I would walk into that surgery knowing exactly who, in my local area or hospital trust, was the right person to be sent to. I would seek out a gastroenterologist who specialises in incontinence and/or issue related to chronic gastric conditions. As I've stated before sadly not all gastroenterologists are up to speed in this very specific area of their own speciality; incontinence is a speciality in its own right.

Here's a sample symptoms diary for you.

| Stool Diary | | | | | | |
|---|---|---|---|---|---|---|
| PLEASE RECORD YOUR STOOL HABIT FOR ONE WEEK: | | | | | | |
| Date | Time of Bowel Movement | Incontinence | Stool Seepage or Staining | Stool Consistency (Type 1-7) | Urgency - unable to postpone BM for more than 15 Minutes | Comments |
| | | Yes/No | Yes/No | See Below | Yes/No | |
| | | | | | | |
| | | | | | | |
| | | | | | | |
| | | | | | | |
| | | | | | | |
| | | | | | | |
| | | | | | | |
| | | | | | | |
| | | | | | | |

<u>Use the following descriptors for describing stool consistency:</u>

Type 1: **Separate hard lumps.** ▪ Type 2: **Sausage shaped but lumpy.** ▪ Type 3: **Like a sausage but with cracks on its surface.** ▪ Type 4: Like a sausage or snake, smooth and soft. ▪ Type 5: **Soft blobs with clear-cut edges (passed easily).**
▪ Type 6: **Fluffy pieces with ragged edges, a mushy stool.** ▪ Type 7: **Watery.**

*Make sure you understand each other – agree on the language…*

# Bristol Stool Chart

Information is power – confusion is chaos.

We've all been in situations where we've had conversations with people and discovered that we were completely misunderstanding each other. This is usually because we weren't using the same baseline of language. Sometimes these situations can be amusing or even hysterical but when it comes to faecal incontinence it would be far from that. Getting your problem understood is likely to be one of the most important things you'll do in your life so there is no room for error.

Doctors use the Bristol Stool Chart to describe the consistency of stools. They do this specifically to avoid the type of confusion I've just described.

Having said that it may have been a long time since your doctor used a Bristol Chart so take this one with you and point!

By using the chart you can establish a base line from which you, and your doctor, can see if you are improving or deteriorating. It will also give them a real understanding of how bad your situation is.

# THE BRISTOL STOOL FORM SCALE

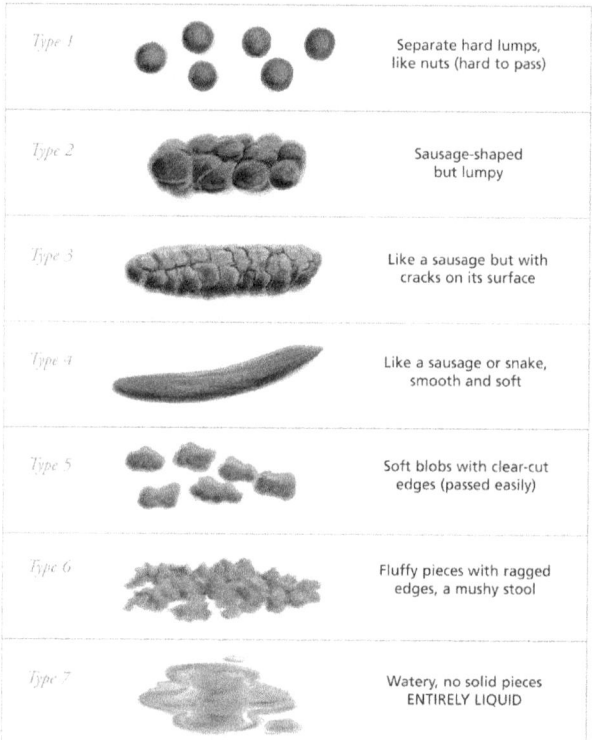

Reproduced with kind permission of Dr KW Heaton,
formerly Reader in Medicine at the University of Bristol.
©2000 produced by Norgine Pharmaceuticals Limited.

*What you should expect from your GP...*

# Your Doctor's Surgery

Quite understandably doctors surgeries differ and some are just better than others. It is practically impossible for all surgeries to offer exactly the same level of care in all fields of medicine. In an attempt to try to provide a guide of the minimum standard required of them the government issues a series of guidelines.

## The NICE clinical guidelines June 2007

Below is an extract from the NICE (National Institute for Health and Care Excellence) guidelines (CG49) June 2007. This may give you an idea of what is required of the practice when you present with symptoms of faecal incontinence. (NB: NICE guidelines operate in the UK only).

If you feel you are not receiving the recommended treatment then discuss that with your doctor.

## Good practice in managing faecal incontinence

People who report or are reported to have faecal incontinence should be offered care to be managed by healthcare professionals who have the relevant skills, training and experience and who work within an integrated continence service.

Because faecal incontinence is a socially stigmatising condition, healthcare professionals should actively yet sensitively enquire about symptoms in high-risk groups

## High-risk groups

- frail older people
- people with loose stools or diarrhoea from any cause
- women following childbirth (especially following third- and fourth- degree obstetric injury)
- people with neurological or spinal disease/injury (for example, spina bifida, stroke, multiple sclerosis, spinal cord injury)
- people with severe cognitive impairment
- people with urinary incontinence
- people with pelvic organ prolapse and/or rectal prolapse
- people who have had colonic resection or anal surgery
- people who have undergone pelvic radiotherapy
- people with perianal soreness, itching or pain
- people with learning disabilities

When assessing faecal incontinence healthcare professionals should:

- be aware that faecal incontinence is a symptom, often with multiple contributory factors for an individual patient
- avoid making simplistic assumptions that causation is related to a single primary diagnosis ('diagnostic overshadowing').

## Baseline assessment and initial management

Healthcare professionals should carry out and record a focused baseline assessment for people with faecal incontinence to identify the contributory factors. This should comprise:

- relevant medical history
- a general examination
- an anorectal examination
- a cognitive assessment, if appropriate.

People with the following conditions should have these addressed with condition-specific interventions before healthcare professionals progress to initial management of faecal incontinence:

- faecal loading
- potentially treatable causes of diarrhoea (for example infective, inflammatory bowel disease and irritable bowel syndrome)
- warning signs for lower gastrointestinal cancer
- rectal prolapse or third-degree haemorrhoids
- acute anal sphincter injury including obstetric and other trauma
- acute disc prolapse/cauda equina syndrome.

Healthcare professionals should address the individual's bowel habit, aiming for ideal stool consistency and satisfactory bowel emptying at a predictable time.

## Specialised management

People who continue to have episodes of faecal incontinence after initial management should be considered for specialised management. This may involve referral to a specialist continence service, which may include:

- pelvic floor muscle training
- bowel retraining
- specialist dietary assessment and management
- biofeedback
- electrical stimulation
- rectal irrigation.

Some of these treatments might not be appropriate for people who are unable to understand and/or comply with instructions

## Long-term management

Healthcare professionals should offer the following to symptomatic people who do not wish to continue with active treatment or who have intractable faecal incontinence:

- advice relating to the preservation of dignity and, where possible, independence
- psychological and emotional support, possibly including referral to counsellors or therapists if it seems likely that people's attitude towards their condition and their ability to manage and cope with faecal incontinence could improve with professional assistance
- at least 6-monthly review of symptoms
- discussion of any other management options (including specialist referral)
- contact details for relevant support groups

- advice on continence products and information about product choice, availability and use
- advice on skin care
- advice on how to talk to friends and family
- strategies such as planning routes for travel to facilitate access to public conveniences, carrying a toilet access card or RADAR key to allow access to 'disabled' toilets in the National Key Scheme.

*Now you know how normal continence functions.*

*You now know what criteria are needed for a diagnosis of IBS*

*You're ready to compile your symptoms information to take with you to your GP*

*You'll already be thinking where you sit on the Bristol Stool Chart*

*and*

*You have some idea of what service your GP's surgery should be offering you.*

*The next step is to understand what tests might be done to determine what is happening in your case.*

# What tests might or should be done

In order to determine exactly what is causing your problem, or to rule out what is not causing it, some tests will need to be undertaken. It is extremely important to pin point the cause of your specific problem because the treatments vary depending on the cause. These test results will also provide a baseline comparison for any future tests of a similar nature. This is important because it may be that there are alternative treatments available and that one may be better for you than another.

The following tests are the most commonly performed. Collectively they will hopefully identify the cause and severity of your symptoms.

## Digital Anal Examination:

This is the simplest of all, yet it can be extremely enlightening.

The procedure is not painful for most people but can be a little uncomfortable and is rather embarrassing.

For me there was often the added embarrassment of knowing, because (as I now know) my internal sphincter was not functioning fully, that the doctor was likely to end up with a soiled finger.

The doctor will usually ask you to lay on your left side and pull your legs up towards your chest to allow clear access to the anus. They will then gently slide a lubricated and gloved finger into the rectum.

This simple examination can turn up such things as irregular surfaces which may suggest there is some scar tissue in the region. The doctor will also ask you to tighten your sphincter so they may assess its strength. Other things that can be observed during this examination are haemorrhoids, anal polyps (if large enough), prolapses, fissures (damaged areas in the external anal sphincter) or even tumours in some cases.

Again with the knowledge I have now, if my GP didn't do this examination on my first visit to them concerning faecal incontinence, or didn't refer me to a specialist, then I would immediately have concerns as to whether they are the right person to see about the problem.

## Stool sample:

Many things can be learnt from our stools which is why your doctor will likely want to have a sample.

You may be given a collection set and asked to do this at home but alternatively you may be asked to go into the toilet then and there. If so you will be given a disposable bed-pan and a small plastic sealed sample pot that contains a little spoon built into the lid.

You have to defecate into the bed-pan and then scoop up a pea sized amount of stool and place it into the sample pot. Once that is done you empty the remaining contents of the bed pan into the toilet and finish your business as usual.

This test is looking for diseases of the digestive tract and in a basic sense is divided into three subgroups.

- Microscopy, to look for bacterium and parasites
- Chemical tests, to look for traces of blood or infection.
- Culture, to work out what bacteria and which antibiotic to use.

## Barium meal

Barium meal examinations are used to search for various diseases or disorders of the digestive system, such things as thinning of the intestinal walls, hernias, constrictions, obstructions, or masses in the oesophagus or stomach. It can also highlight inflammatory diseases of the intestines.

You will be given a drink of a white liquid that contains the chemical (barium sulphate). Barium sulphate shows up on x-rays and allows the radiographer to see your intestines in detail. The drink is usually fruit flavoured and quite thick.

You will be positioned on an x-ray table and may be asked to move into different positions or the doctor may manipulate your stomach with a stick with a half ball on the end. This is done to allow them to see the intestines in different positions.

## Bile acid malabsorption

Bile acid malabsorption is a condition in which bile acid that is produced in the liver is not absorbed back into the body in the normal way. It is a common cause of chronic diarrhoea. It is diagnosed with a SeHCATscan and treated easily. 95% of your bile should be absorbed back into the body as it passes through the small bowel. If it is not absorbed back it passes into the colon and causes diarrhoea.

The test (SeHCAT) involves attending the nuclear medicine department of your hospital where you will be scanned to obtain a baseline reading. You will be given a small pill which contains synthetic bile salt that shows up on the scan. Exactly one week later you attend the clinic again for a second scan. The results of the two scans are compared.

People with normal bile acid function (i.e. it is absorbed back into the body) usually show more than 15% on the scan. If you are not absorbing the acid back into your body then only around 1% – 5% is visible on the scan.

Bile acid malabsorption is treated with the drug, cholestyramine, which you dissolve in a glass of water or juice.

## Endo-Anal ultrasound

Ultra-sound is common practice nowadays particularly in maternity care where it is possible to view the foetus in the womb. This particular ultra-sound is looking to outline the muscles of the anus.

A small finger-like probe is inserted into your bottom. Inside the probe there is a spinning wheel which sends out the sound signal in a circular fashion. The signal then bounces back. The doctor can then see the shape of the muscles of the anal canal and anus on his monitor screen. The muscles can be seen at rest and in motion.

This examination is able to identify problems with the internal and external anal sphincter muscles as well as note any growths in the region.

This simple test, along with the defecography test, were to be my personal life savers. Had these tests been ordered by either of my first two gastroenterologists then I would have been saved much of the horror of my twenty five year ordeal. Why neither of them thought about this piece of the jigsaw will be forever a mystery to me. It is a mystery that should have never been allowed to come about.

## Ano-rectal physiology test

This test measures the pressure within the anal canal. It also takes into account the lower colon (rectum) and the two sphincter's, reaction to that pressure. In other words it is checking if the right signals are being sent, received and implemented by the various muscles involved. The test can determine if there is some damage to the nerves or muscles within.

First you are asked to lay on your left side. A small catheter is inserted which has small holes that contain pressure sensors. This firstly assesses the length of the anal canal and the resting pressure of the internal sphincter. You will then be asked to squeeze as tight as you can and to hold the squeeze during which time the pressure created by the external sphincter is measured. At the same time they will measure the endurance of your sphincter clench. You will also be asked to cough and relax at various times throughout the procedure.

The catheter is removed and another inserted that has a deflated balloon at the top. This is inserted into the rectum, which you will recall is able to stretch to accommodate and store the stool. The volume of the balloon is gradually increased and you will be asked to report any discomfort or pain.

This catheter is removed and a third inserted that is smaller and capable of delivering a weak electric current. The current is gradually increased until you report a slight pain in the region. This tests the nerve stimulation through different nerve pathways.

## Defecography

This test is usually used if constipation is a main symptom and can detect any weakness or incorrect function of the rectum, internal and external sphincter muscles. It will also show up internal hernias and prolapses.

As with the Barium Enema you are filled from the rear with the Barium paste mixture and asked to tell the doctor when you are completely full and feel you need to defecate.

At that point you will move from the trolley onto a commode style toilet seat with a collection bag beneath it. The doctor will ask you to defecate into the collection bag whilst an x-ray film is taken.

The x-ray is taken from the side and the doctor is able to see what your muscles are doing as you tighten, loosen and during defecation of the Barium mixture.

## Endoscopy

Technically an 'endoscopy' is an examination, by endoscope, of any internal organ that is hollow. There are many types of endoscopic examinations but you are most likely to have a gastroscopy, symoidoscopy or colonoscopy. An endoscope is a long tube filled with fibre optic cable. The tube is inserted into the body so that the doctor may see what is happening inside.

# Gastroscopy

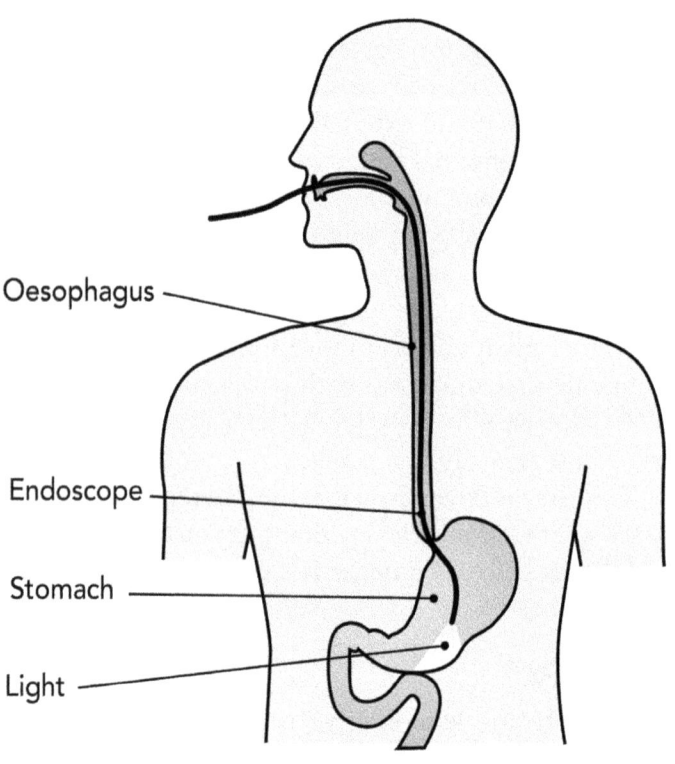

## Gastroscopy

You may have this test done either with, or without, sedation. Whichever way you chose your throat is sprayed with a topical anaesthetic which helps to stop you from gagging as the tube is lowered down through your mouth into your stomach.

The doctor is able to see the surface of the stomach on a monitor and a film is made of the whole procedure. They can also take still pictures of particular areas of interest and a grasping tool can be inserted through the endoscope to take biopsies of the lining of the oesophagus or stomach walls.

In the sigmoidoscopy the scope, which is very similar to the endoscope, is inserted up your bottom as far as the sigmoid colon.

You will be given a bed in an anti-chamber ward and asked to change into a hospital gown that is open at the back. You will then be given an enema some twenty minutes or so prior to the procedure. The enema is usually in a small plastic tube, rather like a small tube of toothpaste. The nurse will lubricate your bottom and then gently insert the enema into you whilst you are lying on your left side with your legs pulled up towards your chest. Once the enema tube is inserted into your anus it is squeezed and the liquid released up into your anus. It is not painful or even uncomfortable as I recall. The chemicals cause your bowel to evacuate after some minutes.

Once you are 'clean' the procedure may begin. The scope is inserted up through the rectum and reaches around as far as the Sigmoid colon. No sedation is required for this procedure. The doctor is able to see any defects and will also look for such things as haemorrhoids, inflammation, polyps or scarring or tumours.

# Sigmoidoscopy

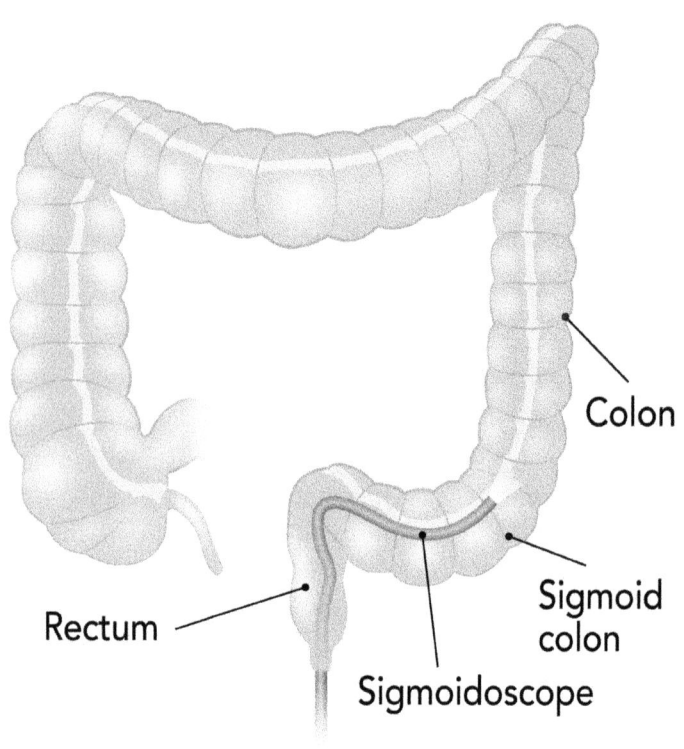

# Colonoscopy

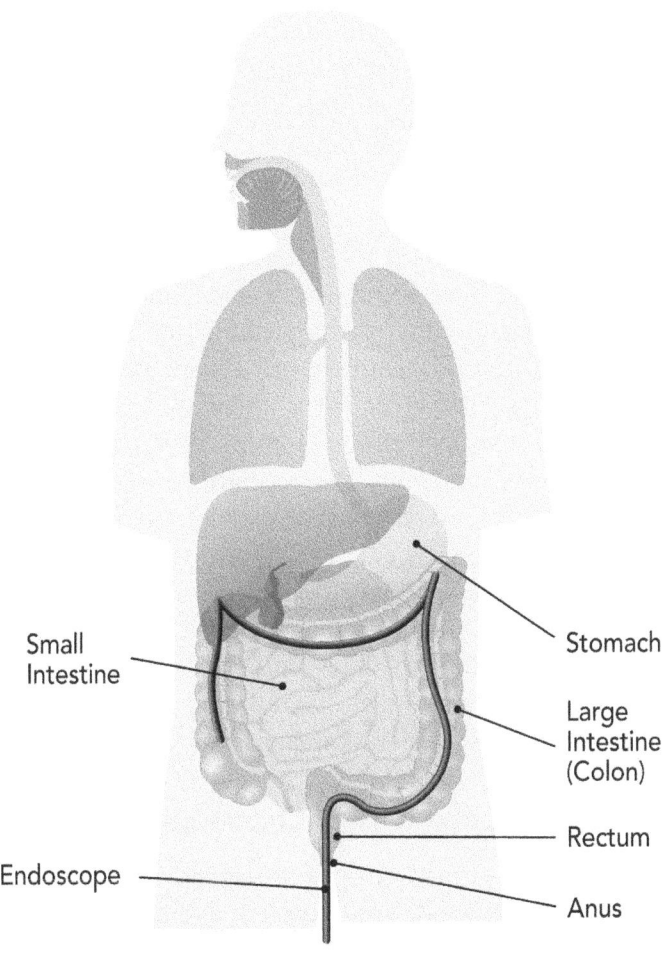

Again, very similar to the endoscopy and sigmoidoscopy a colonoscopy is used to search for defects and abnormalities.

The preparation for this test is however rather unpleasant. The day before you have to drink a preparation of salts that cause you to defecate and defecate and then defecate some more. This mixture must be consumed at set times and you are then unable to eat or drink after a set time.

DO NOT GO TO WORK. STAY AT HOME FOR THIS PREPARATION

Sedation is required for this procedure, as the scope enters the body at some length, but you do not lose consciousness but after the procedure you have little or no memory of it. The entire length of the colon is viewed and biopsies may be taken if there is some area of concern for the doctor. The biopsies do not hurt as the gut does not contain any pain receptor nerves.

You will need to stay in the endoscopy unit for a few hours until the effects of the sedation wear off.

I had some quite heavy discomfort after this procedure. This was caused by the gas that the doctor must insert into the colon to allow himself clear visibility. The discomfort lasted for only a short period of time and was eased with the expulsion of the excess wind.

## CT Colonography (Virtual Colonoscopy)

This is the most modern way of seeing inside the body and specifically inside your bowel and abdomen.

CT colonography involves using a scanner to produce two and three dimensional images of the whole of the large bowel (colon and rectum). The scanner uses x-rays to produce images of a "slice" through a part of the body. This is called Computer Tomography or CT.

During CT colonography, gas will be used to inflate your bowel via a thin flexible tube placed in your back passage. Then the CT scans will be performed with you lying on your back and your front. After the scans, doctors will look at your images for polyps and signs of cancer. If anything unusual is seen on the images, or if further information is needed, you may be offered further tests.

The procedure usually takes around 15-20 minutes. You may have a small tube, called a cannula, inserted into one of the veins in your arm. You will be asked to lie down on the scanner table on your left side. The radiographer will then pass a small flexible tube into your back passage. A muscle relaxant will normally be injected to avoid bowel spasm. Once the radiographer is satisfied with the amount of gas in your bowel, CT scans will be taken with you lying in two positions; usually first on your front or side and then on your back.

## Bowel transit time (for Rapid Gut Transit)

As I mentioned earlier I discovered that I had rapid gut transit by accident after eating some delicious beetroot soup. Interestingly I had thought that beetroot was something that caused my 'problem' to flare up so I usually avoided it like the plague. In fact I'm perfectly fine with it and it was the rapid transit that was the problem, not poor old mister Beetroot. Rapid gut transit is triggered by the endocrine system which for some reason inappropriately releases hormones that speed up the peristalsis throughout the length of the gut. This means that the food is not digested properly and the water is not removed from the faecal matter as it passes through the guts.

Although you could just use beetroot soup yourself, the formal way of testing for this condition is to swallow a capsule containing a dye. After swallowing it you simply wait to see when you notice the red dye in your stools or diarrhoea. You may also measure the time needed for all of the dye to pass through your colon.

NB: although this test is available it is rarely used in clinical practice because it is virtually impossible to establish a baseline reading to compare 'increased' transit to. In other words everyone is different.

## Lactose Intolerance

Lactose is a sugar contained within cow's milk. In order to break down the lactose so that the body can digest it we must produce an enzyme called lactase. Some people are not able to produce this enzyme. This may occur in childhood but is more common in adults and seems to become more prevalent as one ages.

The symptoms are:

- upset stomach
- bloating/flatulence – with associated
- cramps
- diarrhoea
- nausea

(note the symptoms are almost the same as IBS)

The easiest way to check if you are lactose intolerant is to stop eating ANYTHING containing lactose. This may sound easy but you will be surprised how many foods contain lactose. You must read the content of the prepared foods you purchase, any milk (or milk products) should be highlighted in bold (**if in the UK**). Also you must have your thinking cap on when buying food, a croissant for example is packed full of butter yet this will not generally be displayed for the consumer.

One point to note is that lactose is only found in cow's milk so goat's milk products like butter, cheeses and creams are fine. Ewe or buffalo milk cheeses are fine as is any cow's milk cheese that is aged for more than about eight to ten months as the lactose is broken down in the ageing process. Do particularly watch out for mozzarella cheese which can be made from any milk including cow's milk; only consume mozzarella if you are sure it is buffalo milk. Pizza usually uses cow's milk mozzarella as it is a great deal cheaper than buffalo's.

There is a test for lactose intolerance which is the hydrogen breath test. You will be given a drink of a lactose solution and your breath tested to find out how much hydrogen is present. A baseline will have been established before you drink the solution and then the breath tested over a period of a few hours to monitor any changes in the level of hydrogen.

## Blood tests

There are an array of things the doctors test for when you give blood. They will be looking for raised, or lowered levels of certain hormones or enzymes which may alert them to a problem within the body's endocrine system. The endocrine system is the one responsible for the production and release of our hormones.

Blood tests are also able to show up such things as infections or point to conditions such as tumours.

## Coeliac disease – blood test

Coeliac disease is a digestive condition in which one has an adverse reaction to gluten. If a person with coeliac disease consumes gluten they may have a range of reactions including unpleasant smelling diarrhoea, bloating and flatulence, abdominal pain, weight loss and tiredness.

Coeliac disease is an autoimmune condition. The body's defence system starts attacking the healthy tissue because it mistakes elements of the gluten as a threat to the body. The lining of the intestines is damaged by this attack and your ability to absorb nutrients is compromised. The cause of coeliac disease is genetic.

## Urine tests

Urine tests are able to look for infections and excess hormones that are produced and released by the glands in the gut.

You may be asked to have a 24 hour urine sample test which looks for raised hormone levels in the intestines.

Although urine tests may not point directly at a cause of faecal incontinence they help the doctor with the bigger picture of the patient's general state of health and well-being.

Here is a table listing the tests mentioned. Fill in the box to note for your own reference why, or why not, the test was/wasn't done. If you can't fill it all in then you need to find out the answers.

| | | |
|---|---|---|
| Digital Examination | | |
| Stool sample | | |
| Barium meal | | |
| Bile acid malabsorption | | |
| Endo-Anal ultrasound | | |
| Ano-rectal physiology test | | |
| Defecography | | |
| Gastroscopy | | |
| Sigmoidoscopy | | |
| Colonoscopy | | |
| CT Colonography | | |
| Lactose Intolerance | | |
| Blood tests | | |
| Coeliac disease | | |
| Urine tests | | |

*Biofeedback, the daily workout that certainly helped me...*

# Biofeedback

Biofeedback is a relatively new form of treatment that has had excellent results for thousands of people around the world. Putting it in the most basic of terms it is the retraining of your muscles.

As you have seen earlier in the book a state of continence is maintained by a series of intricate interactions, both automatic and conscious, between your muscles and your brain, a 'ballet'. We learn much of our continence 'skills' as we are toilet trained in early childhood. Somehow with faecal incontinence sufferers the body seems to forget some of these skills as the muscles have altered or as the panic attacks develop and overpower us. Biofeedback helps you to take control of your muscles, relearn what they should be doing, and thus aids your continence 'ballet'.

With Biofeedback you learn to be aware of the signals your body is sending back and forth; you learn to be aware of what you are feeling deep within your body. Once you are aware of what you are feeling, and what section of the ballet that refers to, you are able to intervene in the process which can have a very strong and positive impact on your continence.

Think back to the section on normal continence and you will recall that the internal anal sphincter senses a build up of faeces/stool in the rectum and opens for a split second to allow a tiny amount of faeces down the column towards the anus 'a test run'. At the exact same time your external anal sphincter automatically contracts to prevent any leakage from the body whilst your brain decides if you wish to defecate then and there or to wait and go another time.

Babies are not continent because they have not yet learned to clench the external sphincter when they feel the internal one opens. They simply allow the faeces to pass straight through the external sphincter unchecked. Once toilet training starts the child quickly learns to hold back the faeces until they reach the potty.

If you have an issue with the coordination of the two sphincters Biofeedback training will make you aware of the opening of the internal sphincter so that you can secure the external sphincter in time to prevent yourself from having an accident. One way of teaching this is to insert small balloons (the same as the ones used in anorectal physiology test) into the rectum and anus. These balloons are then connected to pressure transducers which record the pressures applied to them by the muscles as they clench.

One balloon is positioned in the rectum, one in the internal sphincter and one at the external sphincter. A polygraph machine, like the lie detector machines on the American police shows, pictorially records what your muscles are doing. The harder you squeeze the higher the tracing goes on the graph paper. You are able to practice the squeezing in order to get the mark on the paper up to the position that your Biofeedback practitioner has set as your desired position.

This process is not only strengthening the sphincter muscle but also teaching you control over it. The normal function of the external sphincter is to instantly contract in response to the opening of the internal sphincter but often in people with faecal incontinence this response is either missing or impaired in some way. Biofeedback training sessions will teach you to once again contract the external sphincter exactly in unison with the opening of the internal sphincter.

At the beginning of the sessions you will be looking at the graph paper and your practitioner will show you what represents the opening of the internal sphincter which they will simulate by inflating the balloon. Once you can recognise this on the paper you will be encouraged to instantly clench your external sphincter. In no time at all most people can do this at great speed.

Once you have become familiar with that technique, and with reaching the required pressure on the clenching of your external sphincter you will be asked to do it again but without the use of the graph paper, just by sensing what you are feeling internally.

You will also be taught to exercise your muscles by holding the contractions for about five or ten seconds before relaxing. You will be asked to do this multiple times in quick succession. This strengthens the muscles which are likely to have weakened over the period of your problem which for some, like me, was years.

Biofeedback session are not long, some taking only about twenty minutes, but in most cases the results are almost instant. You may be asked to return for several sessions over a period of weeks and then for a final top up session after some months. This is done to see if you have successfully mastered the techniques and are applying them as desired.

I learnt two basic biofeedback tricks that I use regularly with great benefit. My wonderful Biofeedback nurse, Ellie Bradshaw, taught me these at our first meeting and this knowledge has been invaluable for me.

The first is simply squeezing my external sphincter while trying to pull it up inside, in other words a really deep internal contraction; I called it the Ellie crunch. All you do is this type of squeeze, has hard as you possibly can, the second you sense something is either happening or is about to happen. I learnt this without even having the balloons inserted. I'm sure that my internal sphincter, because it was not fully functioning, had weakened considerably over the years and that was not helping the 'ballet' at all.

The second trick was using a foot stool for ensuring complete evacuations. Many faecal incontinence sufferers often feel they have not completely emptied themselves. This may be because some faecal material remains in the anal canal or they may have what is know as "funnel-shaped anus". Funnel-shaped anus is a condition in which the weakened muscles structure causes a deformation in the normal shape of the anus that traps the faecal material. If you have great trouble cleaning yourself after an evacuation make sure you mention this to your doctor and biofeedback practitioner. Using a foot stool mimics our natural position for defecation which would be to squat in the bushes. This position assists the evacuations by applying downward pressure from the abdomen. It is most effective and I now have foot stools located at home and at work.

## Correct position for opening your bowels

### Step one
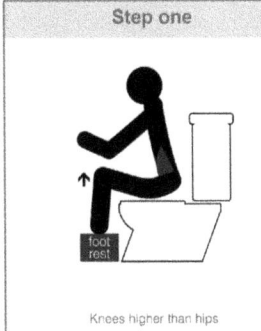
Knees higher than hips

### Step two
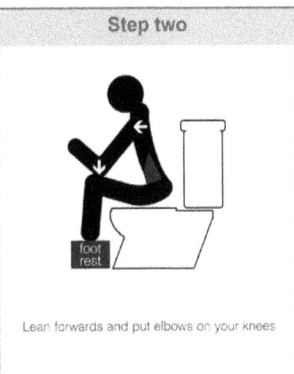
Lean forwards and put elbows on your knees

### Step three
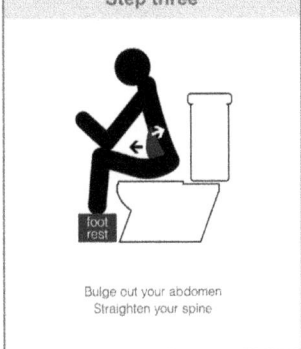
Bulge out your abdomen
Straighten your spine

### Correct position
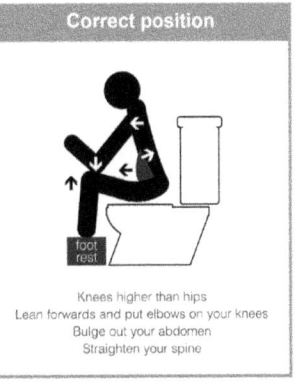
Knees higher than hips
Lean forwards and put elbows on your knees
Bulge out your abdomen
Straighten your spine

It's important to note that everyone is different so if you have Biofeedback training it will be specifically structured for your own situation. I've only touched on two aspects of Biofeedback here so please do research it more thoroughly and discuss it with the practitioner when you meet them.

*Adrenaline, the faecal incontinence sufferer's arch enemy. How bubbles and my cat helped me get over my panic attacks.*

# The emotional and psychological impact

It wasn't until I'd had Harry (my sacral nerve stimulator) implanted and got to grips with the lactose intolerance and rapid gut transit that I realised just how powerful and impactful the effects of adrenaline were on me. I suspect that as it affected me so profoundly then the chances are that it has a similar impact on many others.

Adrenaline is released by our endocrine (hormone) system as part of our fight or flight reflex. It is designed to enable our muscles, and senses, to react and perform at their optimum level instantly. Originally this would have served to protect our lives in the wild should we have come face to face with a predator. Thankfully we tend to get by without the risk of being eaten these days so Adrenaline is not as needed as it once was. It is however an active hormone that must be used up by the body, it cannot simply be reabsorbed back into our systems.

Faecal incontinence sufferers frequently also suffer from panic attacks. Panic attacks are basically the brain telling the body that it is in imminent danger or distress (about to have an accident in the case of faecal incontinence sufferers) so the body responds by instantly releasing adrenaline. As we are not really in 'danger' the adrenaline isn't needed to make us run faster or jump higher so it ends up stimulating the muscles in the stomach and speeding up the function of our intestines. This is why one frequently gets an upset stomach when nervous. I work in the classical music world and I assure you that the toilets are in great demand just before the performers walk on stage.

The complicated thing with panic attacks is that we seem to be able to programme triggers into our subconscious. For me those triggers were often points on the journey to work. Most recently it was a specific corner on the route. A little niggle of fear would strike as I approached the corner and without fail the second I got there my stomach would start to feel the effects of the adrenaline and I'd be on the downhill slide to an accident. Sometimes I'd be able to keep myself going enough to get to work and use the facilities there but more often than not I'd have to stop, park the car illegally, and run to the public loos, or bushes, in the park I passed. If I did make it to work then on occasions I'd not manage to get out of the car park and would relieve myself there. I will give you some helpful hints on preparing yourself for such situations later on in the book.

It's hard to measure exactly how much emotional and psychological impact you suffer as a result of your incontinence as each person reacts differently. I think however it's fair to say that it certainly does affect all of us in some way.

As I've touched on earlier, being in a constant state of heighten awareness is extremely draining. Feeling anxious for extended periods of time increases the level of adrenalin released into the body so that each time adrenaline is released it is released in greater amounts to compensate for your body's familiarity with its effects. Controlling the adrenaline is key for faecal incontinence sufferers and I have found that some simple hypnotic techniques I learnt in my hypnotherapy sessions were extremely effective in calming me, reducing and, in fact, virtually completely alleviating panic attacks.

The hypnosis was not in any way like your stereotypical pocket watching dangling man in a suit or a stage hypnotist counting to three and people falling over left, right and centre. The hypnosis sessions were, in fact, very calm periods in which I almost felt asleep. I never actually felt as if I'd been hypnotised and my psychologist therapist, Val Walters, always said it was more about suggestion than commands. One measure of this calming effect was that on my first session I could hardly concentrate because of the low level laughter I could hear coming from some office staff nearby. It was if they were in the room with me and it had a real impact of my nerves. By the end of my last session I don't recall even noticing them at all.

One of the first things Val had told me to do was to picture in my mind what colour the adrenaline being released into my blood stream was; for me this was yellow. That done, and with eyes closed, I had to take a deep breath and then slowly exhale yellow breath into an imaginary giant bubble; just like blowing bubbles as a child but bigger. The yellow air, she explained, was the adrenaline being exhaled from my body. She would then talk me through the imagery of the yellow air filled bubbles gently floating away into the distance. At the same time she would be drawing my attention to the fact that my body was feeling more calm and relaxed as the adrenaline was being reduced. All of this was done in a very measured, calm and drone-like voice so with few articulations of tone or pitch.

I know it sounds too simple to be true but it worked. I did feel much more relaxed and peaceful. The next step was to implement that out in the real world.

In the period between sessions, when I would feel an attack coming, I would start talking to myself (this bit is my own trick) telling myself:

"this is your brain doing this, not your body, there is no need to panic, just relax, you are fine, your brain is the problem here not your tummy"

After I would say that to myself a few times I would close my eyes and start blowing the bubbles. If I was on the bus I wouldn't perhaps purse my lips as much as I would if in private but I really did exhale slowly and from a deep breath.

With the bubbles mastered we moved on to another hypnotic technique, 'The Special Place'. Val asked me to identify a situation in which I would feel really safe and relaxed. For me that was being all warm and snuggled up in bed with the light peeping through the shutters and with my cat, Phoenix, purring away in a blaze of contentment. These lazy, usually Sunday, mornings seem to be too few and far between but are a real treat.

This additional technique required me to focus on the way being in that situation made me feel. When I'm lucky enough to have these moments the feeling is one of peace and relaxation, almost a dream like state, warm, safe, no pressure, no stress – fabulous!

Once I was able to achieve feeling relaxed in this way I was asked to imagine being in a situation in which the panic would come on. As soon as I could feel the panic coming on I was told to experience the calm of my Special Place. I became really quite good at transporting myself to that bed and the resulting effect on my stomach was palpable. I would have a reduction in fear almost immediately and that in turn would stop the adrenaline from doing its worst. The results were excellent and as I did this more and more my confidence, and belief, in doing it improved quickly and dramatically. I was soon able to reduce the effects of the attacks dramatically and gradually I gained enough control that I could continue on my way without even considering stopping to find a loo.

I'm very much simplifying what took place in the sessions as it would be impossible to even attempt to convey all that Val did (even if I remembered it all) but suffice to say hypnotherapy really worked well for me. I almost never feel in a state of panic, I sleep much better than I have in years, and I am generally more at peace with myself. If you have the opportunity to try it then I urge you to do so.

The sessions I had were about once a week or fortnightly depending on our diaries. Before coming to each session I had to complete a short survey (following) without hesitation; just taking the first 'gut' reaction answer to the question. The questions are from a standard depression scale used in hospitals to gauge one's psychological state. It was interesting to note that my reactions to these questions did change throughout the course of hypnotherapy sessions which showed that I was improving and generally becoming less stressed. You can work out for yourself which of the answers is the winner in each case.

## Hospital Anxiety and Depression Scale **(HADS)**

Please read each item and <u>underline</u> the reply which comes closest to how you have been feeling in the past week. Don't take too long over your replies; your immediate reaction to each item will probably be more accurate than a long thought-out response.

**A.** **I feel tense or 'wound up':**
Most of the time
A lot of the time
From time to time, occasionally
Not at all

**B.** **I still enjoy the things I used to enjoy:**
Definitely as much
Not quite so much
Only a little
Hardly at all

**C.** **I get a sort of frightened feeling as if something awful is about to happen:**
Very definitely and quite badly
Yes, but not too badly
A little but it doesn't worry me.
Not at all

**D.** **I can laugh and see the funny side of things:**
As much as I always could
Not quite so much now
Definitely not so much now
Not at all

**E.** **Worrying thoughts go through my mind:**
A great deal of the time
A lot of the time
From time to time but not too often
Only occasionally

**F.** **I feel cheerful:**
Not at all
Not often
Sometimes
Most of the time

**G.** **I can sit at ease and feel relaxed:**
Definitely
Usually
Not very often
Not at all

**H.** **I feel as if I am slowed down:**
Nearly all the time
Very often
Sometimes
Not at all

**I.** **I get a sort of frightened feeling like 'butterflies' in the stomach:**
Not at all
Occasionally
Quite often
Very often

**J.** I have lost interest in my appearance:
Definitely
I don't take as much care as I should
I may not take as much care
I take just as much care as ever

**K.** I feel restless as if I have to be on the move:
Very much indeed
Quite often
Not very often Not at all

**L.** I look forward with enjoyment to things
As much as ever I did
Rather less than I used to
Definitely less than I used to
Hardly at all

**M.** I get sudden feelings of panic:
Very often indeed
Quite often
Not very often
Not at all

**N.** I can enjoy a good book or radio or TV programme:
Often
Sometimes
Not often
Very seldom

*Hopefully I've given you some useful information on how to go about finding out what is happening with you and how Biofeedback and psychological training might be able to aid your improvement.*

*Now I'm going to talk about ways of coping with FI on a daily basis. Much of this you will have worked out for yourself and there may be some other tricks you might be able to add in to the mix.*

# Coping with 'it' day to day

Over the years we've all worked out ways of trying to cope with the practical problems of dealing with faecal incontinence. I thought I'd list my ways down here for you, along with any ideas I've come across that may be of use to some of you.

## Disposables

Depending on how bad your particular problem is there are a range of disposable products such as ladies' panty liners through to larger more absorbent inserts and full on disposable adult nappies.

I gradually worked my way up through these and found that one of the great side-effects of wearing these is the peace of mind they give you. One of the worst elements of having an accident is the build up to it and the fear and dread surrounding it. If one at least knows that in the worst case you'll have protection enough to allow you, even with soiled pants, to get to a toilet it helps to prevent the panic attacks and anxiety.

There are many products available on the market so look up incontinence products on the internet and you'll soon come across something to suit you. I chose products that folded up small enough for me to carry them in my shoulder bag.

## Taking Imodium

Knowing how to take Imodium changed things very positively for me. I wish I'd been told this years before.

Imodium, (Loperamide), is a wonderfully simple medication that is known as an active drug. This means that it works only when taken and that there are no long term, or hangover, effects. Many people with faecal incontinence will also likely have issues with the consistency of their stools. The runnier the stool, or faecal material, the less able we are of holding it back with the anal sphincters. Loperamide slows down the gut and as a result more water is removed from the material allowing the stools to form in the normal way.

I had always taken Loperamide as the problems were appearing but in reality this was the least effective way of using the drug. The best way is to take the dose about thirty minutes to one hour before food. If you have a consistent problem, like me, then your doctor may suggest that you take the doses regularly before meals. Each person will have a slightly different reaction to Loperamide so you need to do some trial and error to establish what dose works best for you. I now have four before breakfast, three before lunch and one before dinner. This has taken me from a score ranging from six to seven of the Bristol Stool Chart to a healthy, dare I say almost normal, three!

Using Loperamide to keep the stools in a solid form will allow the rectum and anus to function to the best of their ability depending on your personal situation.

This will also aid your confidence and help to prevent the panic attacks and feelings of incomplete evacuation. Note that Loperamide is often available in supermarkets at a considerably reduced price compared with the branded product.

## Aisle Seats

Making sure you have an aisle seat on planes, trains, theatres etc helps a little as you know you can jump up at any point should you need to dash to the loo.

I travel a great deal by plane for my work and always go to some lengths to ensure that I have an aisle seat as close to the front toilets as possible. The two reasons for this are: firstly, less people use the front loos and secondly you can get off the plane sooner in order to be near the terminal toilets. With European airlines sitting at the front usually costs more money (business class) so, if I'm not in the posh bit, I always carry an IBS card that I show to the cabin crew when I board. The card explains that I have a non-infectious condition that necessitates that I need to have immediate access to a toilet. So far all of the cabin crew I have come in contact with have been supportive and most helpful by allowing me to use the business class section toilet. If I'm sitting towards the rear of the plane then I would always go further back to be close to the toilets.

The cards are available through various IBS sites. For example.

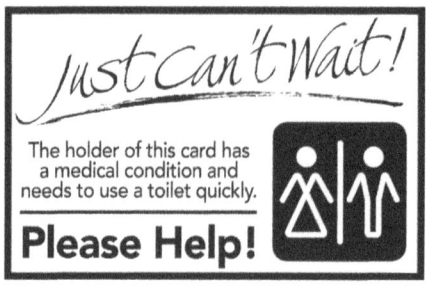

## Radar Keys

Radar keys are a standard key used on most locked disabled toilets in the UK. These keys are available to disabled persons but they are also available on the internet for just a few pounds.

I had a quick look on the internet and found one company claiming:

*"Our Disabled toilet keys fit the Wellington lock that is used by Radar and the National Key Scheme, helping you access the 7000 disabled toilets across the UK. We sell keys with a larger head for those with limited dexterity and a standard shaped key."*

Rather annoyingly I didn't know about this key until researching for this book so hopefully this one may give you a head-start.

## Apps

With the development of smart phones wonderful toilet finding apps are readily available. For any of you who are not familiar with smart phones then in simple terms what these application do is to work out where you are in the world and then it shows you on a map where the nearest toilets are. These apps vary but many of them now include toilets that users have added themselves. This is marvellous as you get to find the hidden toilets that otherwise you may not have seen.

Some of these apps will actually give you directions like a sat nav system does in your car. This really is technology coming to our aide.

## Your bag of goodies

Most of you will have already worked this one out for yourselves. In short you need to have everything with you that you might need to get yourself out of trouble or cleaned up after an accident.

My bag contained (how I love now using past tense) extra incontinence pad(s), a plastic bag to dispose of a soiled one in, wet wipes and tissue paper, wind-ease pills, spare (thin) trousers and underpants, coins for use in automated loos and extra Imodium and the anti-depressants (I was on them then).

I was on business in Japan when the Icelandic volcano erupted in 2010 and was stuck there for an extra five days. I got back to the UK with only one anti-depressant pill left so I learnt then to always take enough spare pills, of whichever medication I need, with me to cover any unexpected delays.

## Plan your journey

If you're going out of your normal area it's wise to plan which route you'll take and try to work out where the loos are on the way. Now days with Google maps and street view it is much easier to do this. Knowing where the pubs and fast food places are will help you to avoid a panic attack and just make the whole journey less stressful.

Before we had these modern aides I would frequently go for a dummy run in advance of these trips to get the lay of the land and make a mental map of the loos.

## Letting others know

If you have someone you feel you can speak with about your problem I would urge you to do so. The old adage 'a problem shared is a problem halved' may not be quite accurate but I assure you when I decided to tell my friends it felt like a huge weight had been lifted from my shoulders. Needing INSTANT access to a loo while out was no longer a matter of having to fabricate some story to cover myself. My friends were understanding and supportive – I wish now I'd been honest with them years before.

On a side note, I do feel it is harder for us boys with faecal incontinence as you girls are allowed to disappear off to the loo whenever the will takes you. No one would ever question you as to why you need to go again, or why were you so long (time for a little confession here – on a lot more than one occasion I've used the ladies' loos! they're cleaner and there are more cubicles).

But seriously if you are able to speak with someone about this you will feel much better and it may give you the strength to get yourself thoroughly investigated. Just finding out what the problem is will often make a big difference.

## Tinted windows in the car

If you have the possibility to have a car with tinted windows do it ! Although I couldn't have afforded it in the earlier days I now drive a larger car that has room in the back that, if really needed can double as porta-cabin loo. The rear section windows are heavily tinted and no one can see in. For the front window you could buy one of those sun blocking 'cardboard pull across things', side windows – baby shops sell pull down blinds. Bingo! your own private bathroom.

Now this leads me on to something I've just discovered while writing this book. It's amazing and I'm gutted I didn't know about it years ago.

Introducing...

## Bog in a bag

This is essential frontline kit. It's a black plastic bag containing a gel pad that absorbs 700mls of liquid. You can use it in conjunction with a collapsing stool (sold separately) but equally you can simply squat and get on with it.

As you use it the gel pad expands and you dispose of it all in any normal bin. Suddenly there's no absolute need to find a loo instantly. You could easily use this bag in a cupboard or any private room. If I still had my faecal incontinence I would definitely not go anywhere with out one of these angels! Again having this with you will really reduce the number of panic attacks you'll suffer – it's amazing.

Look up 'Bog In a Bag' on Amazon.

*Some people have issues with certain foods...*

# Dietary issues

As I've made very clear faecal incontinence is not caused by IBS, equally so it is not caused by dietary problems but they can possibly be playing a role in your problem as a whole.

Again, for me, lactose intolerance was exacerbating my situation because the malfunctioning internal sphincter had no chance of holding back diarrhoea that was under pressure.

First of all if you think that food may be a contributing factor for you then keep a food diary and start noting any commonalities against your symptoms. If there is an issue you should start to see a pattern appear quite quickly.

Here are a few things to look up and look out for and to test yourself for if you are concerned.

Nightshade vegetables are a group of vegetables that were, relatively recently (400 years ago), introduced into our Western diet. Some people do not tolerate the alkaloids found in nightshade vegetables and this may cause many symptoms including upset stomach.

Nightshades (a short list):

- Chili peppers
- Cayenne

- Aubergine/Egg Plant
- Jalapeno peppers
- Paprika
- Pimentos
- Potatoes (not sweet potatoes)

If you think these are causing you an issue then please do more research as this list is in no way exhaustive. NB: there are also some fruits that contain the same alkaloids.

### Gluten

I mentioned coeliacs disease in the section on blood test.

Some people are not able to digest gluten which is found in:

- wheat,
- barley
- rye.
- It may also be contained in many pre-packed products such as:

- pasta
- cakes
- breakfast cereals
- most types of bread
- certain sauces
- ready meals

Coeliacs disease causes:

- diarrhoea, which may smell particularly unpleasant
- bloating and flatulence (passing wind)

- abdominal pain
- weight loss
- feeling tired all the time as a result of malnutrition (not getting enough nutrients from food)

Below is an interesting extract from a paper by Maria I. Vazquez-Roque of the Mayo Clinic. In short it shows that there is a link between gluten and diarrhoea predominate IBS.

## Gluten-free diet for IBS

*Most people who suffer from IBS notice a relationship between specific dietary products and severity of their symptoms and yet there is little scientific evidence for specific dietary restrictions in IBS. That is until recently. A group of researchers from the Mayo clinic explored the relationship between gluten intake and symptoms. They recruited people with diarrhoea predominant IBS and in whom coeliac disease (gluten sensitivity) was excluded by blood tests and in some cases by small bowel biopsies. The study compared the effect of a gluten free diet and a gluten containing diet on symptoms, gut motility and permeability. The results were also analysed according to those who had a genetic predisposition to coeliac disease (HLA DQ4/8) and those who did not. After a four week diet, the group on a gluten free diet experienced less diarrhoea compared with those on gluten containing diet. Interestingly, the improvement was more noticeable in those with the genetic predisposition to coeliac. The gluten containing diet was associated with increased permeability in the small bowel. This is the first study which shows an improvement in IBS with a gluten free diet and a plausible underlying explanation for the improvement i.e. dietary gluten was linked with increased permeability particularly in those with coeliac genetic predisposition. In clinical practice it is unlikely that genotype will be requested to define those who may show greatest response however the results support the approach that a trial with gluten free diet should be attempted in patients presenting with diarrhoea predominant IBS.*

There is a great deal of information available on the internet for digestive problems that are food related so do look into this more if you feel food may be having an impact on you.

*If you are one of the people with a malfunctioning or damaged internal sphincter then maybe 'Harry' is the 'man' for you...*

# Sacral Nerve Stimulation: living with Harry

If, like me, you have a malfunction of, or damage to, the internal anal sphincter then 'Harry' may be for you.

Basically the InterStim is a pacemaker that helps to regulate the messages that the muscles send to the brain. In my experience it is fair to say that at this stage it is not known exactly how Harry works but it is known that he does work.

In my case he has made an incredible difference to me and my entire life. Before the implant I was managing from day-to-day and would not be able to accept spontaneous social or work events, that would have been simply too risky. Everything had to be planned ahead, business meetings and trips all had to be planned with great care.

This had come to a head in relation to work meetings about six months before Harry came along. I was chairing a meeting of our board of directors with experts from a particular company. The meeting was in the offices of the external company and naturally I started with the urgency and fear which turned into a full blown panic attack. Trouble was that I was in charge of the whole room and couldn't just get up and go to the loo. I'd noted where the loos were of course but I was leading the meeting, everyone was focused on me. Finally I had no option other than to pause the meeting and excuse myself; the embarrassment was overwhelming. I did manage to get out of there without a full on accident but the stress was incredible and I was exhausted and deeply depressed that evening.

The next morning I emailed the entire board of directors and explained that my 'IBS' had become so bad that off-site meetings were no longer an option. This was extremely embarrassing for a young man (forties) especially as I was the one in charge of the whole show, in charge but I couldn't be away from a toilet, just like a baby.

Damage to the internal sphincter is most common in women who have suffered some injury to it during childbirth. Unfortunately they often do not know they have been damaged. If they knew they would be a big step ahead when their faecal incontinence starts.

Malfunctioning sphincters are very rare and I guess being a male put me at a disadvantage and is probably an underlying reason that it took so long for the appropriate tests to be done that determined that my internal sphincter was thin in one section. No one knows why it is thin in that section and operations to repair such conditions are rarely successful in the long term so not usually considered as an option.

Day-to-day living with Harry is no trouble at all. He comes with a remote control unit so that I can adjust the electric pulse he omits up and down as needed but sometimes I don't adjust him for days or even weeks. I hardly feel the pulse he gives out. In the beginning I was adjusting him up and down all the time but that has reduced as my confidence and belief in him has improved.

If your tests show that you have some issue with your internal sphincter then your doctor should consider whether Harry is right for you.

Below is some information from the website for InterStim.

**What Is InterStim™ Therapy?**

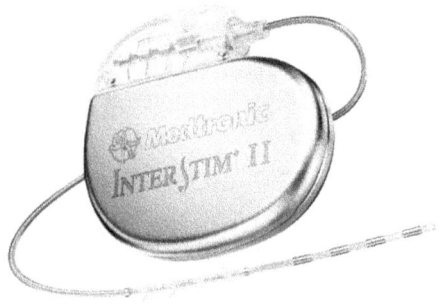

*The InterStim II neurostimulator for overactive bladder, urinary retention, faecal incontinence and constipation.*

*With sacral neuromodulation InterStim II, a small device, just a little bit bigger than a 2 euro coin, is surgically implanted to stimulate your sacral nerves with mild electrical pulses. The sacral nerves control your bladder and bowel. InterStim therapy is used to treat overactive bladder, urinary retention, faecal incontinence and constipation. If you have not experienced success with more standard treatments, this reversible treatment may be a good option for you.*

## How it works

*The sacral nerves control your bladder, your bowel, your rectum and the muscles related to urinary and anal functions. By stimulating these nerves with a mild electric current, the neurostimulator helps your bowel, rectum and bladder to work as they should.*

## About the InterStim Therapy system

*The InterStim Therapy system consists of:*

- *The implantable neurostimulator, which is like a pacemaker, implanted under the skin*
- *A thin wire that carries the mild electrical pulses to the nerves controlling the pelvic floor, including the bowel and the bladder*
- *A hand-held patient programmer that allows you to adjust the strength of the stimulation and to turn the system on or off.*

*Sacral neuromodulation may help you to regain control and avoid the embarrassment and frustration of bladder and bowel problems.*

# Epilogue

The purpose of this book is to prevent some of you from getting stuck in the IBS black hole. I wanted to do this by empowering you with enough knowledge so that you can play an active part in the diagnosis and treatment of your specific problem.

I hope that I have managed to impart things well enough so that you now have an understanding of what should be happening within your body to enable you to maintain continence. That knowledge should give you at least some clues as to what may be contributing to your inability to maintain it.

By knowing what tests should or might be suggested you will be able to take a proactive role in understanding your condition and getting to grips with finding the best solution for you.

I do think it's import to understand that although some of you will hopefully be helped to live a 'normal' life again we, as a group, must accept that we are not 'normal'. We are a group of people that are faecally incontinent and live our lives by controlling the symptoms of our relevant condition.

I hope to have shown you some pathways that will guide you to finding the right sort of help both for the medical and physiological aspects as well as getting over any of the psychological impacts that this dreadful condition imposes on us.

This book is not here to replace your doctor nor is it in anyway a medical treatment guide. Please use it as a friend and support; remember YOU ARE NOT ALONE.

\*\*\*\*\*\*\*\*\*\*\*\*\*\*\*\*\*\*\*\*\*\*\*\*

And sadly a very depressing PS:

Just as I finished this book a programme ran on the TV which was about GP's. It was a fly-on-the-wall type programme showing conversations between the doctors and their patients.

A poor man in his sixties was seen by his GP for what, based on the conversation, appeared to have been the third time. He had developed faecal incontinence in recent months and during this particular visit described two 'new' episodes of catastrophic faecal incontinence that had occurred since his last appointment; one was in his kitchen at home and the other in a local shopping centre. As he described it, the embarrassment and shame he and his wife suffered, he welled with tears. It was awful to see a delightful and gentle man, who should be enjoying his life, reduced to tears; I found myself deeply moved for him.

He reiterated to the doctor that he was expelling faeces so powerfully that it was spraying, not only the toilet basin, but him. He described that at best it was pencil like in appearance but usually is was diarrhoea under pressure and that he simply could not hold it in no matter when or where he was.

The doctor had done standard blood tests, he read them out from the screen, there was no mention of bile malabsorption or coeliac. However the thing that made me really shudder was that he then confidently proclaimed 'well I think I better do a digital examination of your back passage'. After an unremarkable digital examination the man was sent away and told to come back in three months if it had not calmed down. I was speechless.

This was at least the man's third visit, he was suffering terribly yet clearly not getting investigated properly. Viewing this with the knowledge I have now I see that the doctor had no idea what was going on. More worrying though was the fact that he did not acknowledge that he did not have the necessary knowledge and pass the patient on to a suitably qualified specialist.

Clearly some things haven't changed in the twenty odd years since I experienced this sort of slack medical practice. This made me realise that this book is long overdue.

www.ingramcontent.com/pod-product-compliance
Ingram Content Group UK Ltd.
Pitfield, Milton Keynes, MK11 3LW, UK
UKHW022210230426
12048UKWH00016BA/764